My Twin Pregnancy Week by Week:

The Ultimate Planner for Moms Expecting Twins

Christina Baglivi Tinglof

This planner belongs

to

Jacque Whited

ISBN-13: 978-1503045163
ISBN-10: 1503045161

Visit the author's website, **Talk About Twins,**
for the free printable downloads mentioned in this book:

http://christinabaglivitinglof.com/free-downloads

Table of Contents

Introduction   7

My Twin Pregnancy Fact Sheet   11

My Twin Pregnancy To-Do List   13

MY FIRST TRIMESTER   17

Week 6 Stat Sheet   19
  Choosing a Health-Care Provider   20

Week 7 Stat Sheet   21
  Sample Menu for Moms Expecting Twins   22

Week 8 Stat Sheet   25
  Twin Pregnancy Food Diary   26
  My Food Diary Notes   27
  My Daily Food Diary   28

Week 9 Stat Sheet   29
  My Twins' Ultrasound Photos   30

Week 10 Stat Sheet   31
  Baby Budget Checklist   32

Week 11 Stat Sheet   35

My Twin Pregnancy Journal   36

Week 12 Stat Sheet   37

My Latest Test Results   38

MY SECOND TRIMESTER   39

Week 13 Stat Sheet   41

Maternity Clothes Shopping Tips   42

Maternity Clothes Wish List   43

Maternity Clothes Shopping Notes   44

Week 14 Stat Sheet   45

My Twin Nursery Planning Graph   46

My Twin Nursery Design Ideas   47

Twin Nursery Furniture Checklist   49

My Twin Nursery Shopping Notes   50

Week 15 Stat Sheet   51

My Twin Pregnancy Journal   52

Week 16 Stat Sheet   53

My Twins' Ultrasound Photos   54

Week 17 Stat Sheet   57

My Twin Baby Shower   58

Twin Registry "Must Haves"   59

Week 18 Stat Sheet   61

My Latest Test Results   62

Week 19 Stat Sheet   63
Tips to Choosing a Childbirth Class   64

Week 20 Stat Sheet   65
Tips to Naming Twins   66
Possible Twin Baby Names   67

Week 21 Stat Sheet   69
Know the Signs of Preeclampsia   70

Week 22 Stat Sheet   71
Car Seat Comparison Chart   72

Week 23 Stat Sheet   73
Know the Signs of Preterm Labor   74

Week 24 Stat Sheet   75
My Latest Test Results   76

Week 25 Stat Sheet   77
Double Stroller Comparison Chart   78

Week 26 Stat Sheet   79
My Twins' Ultrasound Photos   80

Week 27 Stat Sheet   81
My Twin Pregnancy Journal   82

MY THIRD TRIMESTER   83

Week 28 Stat Sheet   85
My Latest Test Results   86

Week 29 Stat Sheet   87

    My Post Twins Help Schedule   *88*

Week 30 Stat Sheet   89

    My Twin Pregnancy Journal   90

Week 31 Stat Sheet   93

    My Twin Pregnancy Journal   94

Week 32 Stat Sheet   95

    My Latest Test Results   96

Week 33 Stat Sheet   97

    Twin Layette Checklist   98

Week 34 Stat Sheet   101

    My Twins' Birth Announcement Ideas   102

Week 35 Stat Sheet   103

    My Baby Shower Memories   104

Week 36 Stat Sheet   107

    Daily Feeding and Diapering Chart   108

Week 37 Stat Sheet   109

    My Twin Pregnancy Journal   110

MY NEWBORN TWINS   111

My Newborn Twins' Stat Sheet   113

    My Newborn Twins' Footprints   115

    Newborn Notes   116

Introduction

Expecting twins? That is so exciting! But it is also a bit overwhelming and a little scary, isn't it? You have heard the stories, I am sure, of how you will need to take extra special care of yourself, more so than if you were expecting just one baby. For instance, you will need to gain a bit more weight than you first thought, concentrating on getting enough protein in your diet. (Appropriate weight gain in a twin pregnancy is your *Number One* defense against preterm labor and delivery.) You will also need to slow down, cutting back dramatically on your exercise regimen as physical activity may increase the odds of preterm labor. And get ready for plenty of doctor visits, too, as you are going to be monitored more carefully, undergoing more tests than if you were expecting a single baby. But the payoff will all be worth it. Just imagine — two babies to love and nurture. Two siblings who will grow up together, establishing a bond that will last throughout their lives. How cool is that? Yes, it is exciting expecting twins but it is also a lot of work. But don't worry, you picked up the right book to help you through this journey of a lifetime.

MY TWIN PREGNANCY WEEK BY WEEK

My Twin Pregnancy Week by Week is a planner and journal designed with you in mind — the mom expecting twins. Unlike pregnancy planners and journals geared toward women pregnant with just a single child (or 'singleton,' as we like to say), *My Twin Pregnancy Week by Week* zeroes in on your special needs, your unique circumstances. Everything in this planner focuses a multiple pregnancy, systematically taking you through all nine months, helping you not only get your body in optimal shape, but also your home and family organized and ready for the arrival of twins.

For instance, the planner tracks your weekly weight gain, pregnancy symptoms, questions to ask your doctor and your prenatal test results. Checklists throughout the book help you stay on track with your diet, your baby budget, your maternity clothes shopping, your nursery room planning, and your twin layette. There is also plenty of room to display photos of your growing double bump as well as ultrasound photos of your twin babies. And finally, there's plenty of opportunity to write down your thoughts and feelings during this exciting time in your life in the journal sections of the book.

But most importantly, *My Twin Pregnancy Week By Week* is a planner for the busy mom-to-be who likes to have lots of information, organizational charts, and to-do lists right at her fingertips.

HOW TO USE THIS PLANNER

Organized into chapters (or weeks), *My Twin Pregnancy Week by Week* is completely user-friendly. To coincide with a typical twin pregnancy, the planner begins at Week Six, the time when many moms learn that they are carrying twins (but if you first learn the news at Week Eight or even Week Ten, it is no big deal, just start tracking your progress from that point on), and concludes with Week 37. Why Week 37, a whole three weeks earlier than the standard pregnancy planner? Remember that yours is a special pregnancy, one where research has now shown that the optimal time for delivery is Week 37, not Week 40. Most, but not all, obstetricians now recommend that their patients deliver if and when they reach Week 37.

The beginning of the planner has a *Fact Sheet*, a ledger where you can notate important names and numbers of all your doctors such as your obstetrician, perinatologist (a doctor who specializes in multiple pregnancies), and doula or birthing coach. You can input your important health data too, such as your due date, your pre-pregnancy weight and your weight-gain goal. Next up is a good old-fashioned checklist so you can quickly see at a glance all that needs to be accomplished before your babies make their appearance (think:

checking on health insurance coverage, signing up for childbirth classes, choosing two names that go together well, organizing and preparing the nursery — all different for a mom pregnant with twins).

Then the planner takes you week by week through your pregnancy alerting you to specific details to a twin pregnancy as they occur. For instance, in Week 12, the planner reminds you to ask your doctor for a chorionicity scan to determine if your twins share a placenta (a risk factor for twin-to-twin transfusion syndrome, a dangerous condition that affects approximately 15 percent of identical twins with a common placenta). There are plenty of useful charts included in *My Twin Pregnancy Week by Week* as well. For instance, in Week 8, you will find a *Twin Pregnancy Food Diary* so you can accurately track your daily caloric and protein intake — a must for a healthy pregnancy. A *Twin Nursery Planning Graph* is tucked into Week 14 or, take advantage of the *Double Stroller Comparison Chart* while shopping for baby equipment (Week 25), as the stroller is by far the most important purchase you will make. There is a *Twin Layette Checklist* in Week 33, and even a *Daily Feeding and Diapering Chart* (Week 36) to help you keep your head above water that first crazy month after your babies arrive. (All of these charts are also available to download for free at my website, *Talk About Twins,* http://christinabaglivitinglof.com/free-downloads.)

And although this planner focuses on organization, you will find many medical tidbits peppered throughout the planner with **Did You Know,** facts that are specific to a twin pregnancy that will help you thrive, and **Pregnancy Tips,** little bits of wisdom and advice to help make your pregnancy a healthy one. The book culminates with the chapter, *My Newborn Twins,* where you can post your babies' first photos, their footprints, notate the time they were born, and record each twin's height and weight.

AND SO THE JOURNEY BEGINS

Carry this planner with you — drop it in your handbag; keep it in your briefcase. This way you will be ready to accurately track your weight, blood pressure, and test results every time you visit your obstetrician. But best of all, once your babies are born, this planner will become a treasured keepsake for years to come, one that you will want to someday share with your twins.

MY TWIN PREGNANCY

Fact Sheet

THE JOURNEY BEGINS

Today's date: *Oct 10, 2016*

This is my *1st* pregnancy.

My due date is *April 14, 2017*

My pre-pregnancy weight: *170*

My twin pregnancy weight goal: _____

My pre-pregnancy waist (inches): _____

My pre-pregnancy bust size (inches): *38*

My pre-pregnancy blood pressure: _____

My Obstetrician:

Lilibird Pichardo
Name

_____
Address

_____
Office Hours

_____
Phone

_____
Email

Piedmont Fayette
Hospital Affiliation

My Perinatologist/Fetal Specialist:

_____
Name

_____
Address

_____
Phone

_____
Email

Doula/Birthing Coach:

_____
Name

_____
Address

_____
Phone

_____
Email

Hospital Where I Will Deliver:

Piedmont Fayette
Name

_____
Address

_____
Phone

_____
Scheduled Hospital Tour Date

My Twins' Pediatrician:

_____
Name

_____
Address

_____
Phone

_____
Email

My Childbirth Class:

_____
Where

_____
Day and Time

_____
Date of First Class

My Health Insurance Information:

_____
Company Name

_____
Phone

_____
Group Number & Policy Number

_____
Claims Address

To-Do List

Here is the mother of all to-do lists—everything you will need to accomplish by Week 37, your estimated week of delivery. Items are in chronological order. Simply check off each one as you complete the task!

First Trimester: Weeks 6 to 12

☑ Begin taking prenatal vitamins.

☑ Interview and choose obstetrician and/or perinatologist. Make my first appointment.

☑ Schedule a checkup with dentist as teeth and gums are more vulnerable during pregnancy.

☑ Calendar a weekly reminder in my smartphone to take a Double Bump Selfie.

☐ Keep a food diary, shooting for a minimum of 3,000 calories and 130 grams of protein each day.

☑ Read up on how to have a healthy twin pregnancy.

☑ Review health insurance coverage.

☐ Set up a baby budget. Start a separate savings account for post-baby expenses. Add to it weekly.

☑ Announce my pregnancy to family and friends.

☐ Discuss "what-if" scenarios with my practitioner ("What if" I go into preterm labor? "What if" I go past my estimated due date EDD?) as every doctor follows a different protocol.

☐ Ask my physician for a *chorionicity scan* to determine if my twins share a single placenta. If they do, my *monochorionic pregnancy* should be monitored much more closely to watch for signs of *twin-to-twin transfusion syndrome (TTTS)*.

Second Trimester: Weeks 13 to 27

- [ ] Plan a date night.

- [ ] Take stock of my wardrobe and shop for essential maternity clothes, especially a good nursing bra.

- [ ] Review my employer's maternity leave policy then schedule a meeting with my boss to inform her about my pregnancy.

- [x] Gather nursery design ideas online from Pinterest and Project Nursery.

- [ ] Scope out a private spot at work where I can take several 15-minute breaks during the day.

- [x] Start brainstorming baby names.

- [ ] Begin to prepare older siblings for the arrival of twins.

- [ ] Consult veterinarian or trainer about preparing pets for arrival of twins.

- [ ] Research and then purchase two, rear-facing car seats.

- [ ] Create a birth plan.

- [ ] Enroll in childbirth classes beginning no later than Week 24 (but shoot for Week 20).

- [ ] Enroll in infant CPR class.

- [ ] Research and then purchase a double stroller.

- [ ] Set up twin nursery. Assemble crib and other baby gear.

- [ ] Discuss delivery options with my physician. Natural birth, vaginal birth, planned cesarean? It will all depend on my babies' "presentation," or position in the uterus.

- [ ] Investigate cord blood banking.

- [ ] Consider going on maternity leave early resting until the birth of my babies. If I do, investigate Disability Insurance to help offset lost wages.

- [ ] Create a baby registry. Tell the hostess of my baby shower that I would like the party between Week 24 to 28 just in case my babies show up early.

Third Trimester: Weeks 28 to 37

- [ ] Plan a date night.

- [ ] Memorize the warning signs of preterm labor. I will not hesitate to call my doctor if I have a concern.

- [ ] Meet with lactation consultant for tips and best practices on breastfeeding.

- [ ] Investigate childcare options. Weigh the cost of childcare against staying home full time.

- [ ] Interview and choose a pediatrician.

- [ ] Enroll older children in New Brother/New Sister class at hospital where I will be delivering my twins.

- [ ] Start recruiting family and friends to help once the babies are home. Set up a tentative help schedule.

- [ ] Decide on a trusted family member who will stay the night with my children when you go into labor.

- [ ] Arrange for someone to care for my pets and look after my home while I'm in the hospital.

- [ ] Choose a birth announcement. Print address labels. Buy stamps.

- [ ] Start cooking and freezing one-pot meals like stew, chili, lasagna.

- [ ] Stock up on pantry and toiletry items. (Think: canned goods, diapers in a variety of sizes and toilet paper.)

- [ ] Look ahead six months for upcoming birthdays and holidays. If necessary, go shopping for gifts and cards.

- [ ] Sign up for online shopping like Amazon Mom so I have front-door delivery. Stockpile take-out menus from local restaurants, especially from those that deliver.

- [ ] Fill in missing items from twin layette.

- [ ] Put the final touches on the nursery. Wash and hang baby clothing.

- [ ] If finances permit, hire a housekeeper to deep clean my home. (Or, at least get my carpets cleaned.)

- [ ] Schedule a hair appointment.

- [ ] Plan a date with older child/children. Do something special that he/she wants to do.

- [ ] Think of a system for telling newborns apart.

- [ ] Make sure cellphones and digital camera batteries are charged.
- [ ] Pay bills for the next month.
- [ ] Install infant seats in the car.
- [ ] Pack my hospital bag.

Once the Babies Arrive (or the Fourth Trimester)

- [ ] Apply for social security numbers for babies. (This can be done in the hospital when I fill out birth certificate information.)
- [ ] Review our will and assign a guardian to our babies. Update life insurance.
- [ ] Send out baby announcements.
- [ ] Schedule babies' first photography session.
- [ ] Write thank-you notes for all baby gifts.
- [ ] Open two 529 College Savings Plans to save for babies' college education. (Babies will need social security numbers.)
- [ ] Join my local Mothers of Twins club. (Find my local chapter at nomotc.org.)

Notes:

_____

_____

_____

_____

_____

My First Trimester

Week 6

Place
My Baby-Bump
Photo here

31 WEEKS TO GO

Today's date: _____

My weight: _____

Pounds gained this week: _____

Pounds to go to reach my goal: _____

My growing waistline in inches: _____

My growing bust size in inches: _____

Questions to ask my doctor:

_____
_____
_____
_____
_____

My pregnancy symptoms:

_____
_____
_____
_____
_____

My Energy Level (circle one):   1   2   3   4   5

Choosing a
Health-Care Provider

Many women expecting twins, especially older moms-to-be, choose to be in the care of a perinatologist (a.k.a. maternal-fetal medicine specialist), a board-certified physician who is well versed in high-risk pregnancies. (And, yes, if you are expecting twins, you are considered high risk regardless of your age, even if you do not experience any complications.) These doctors work with hospitals with Level III neonatal intensive-care units (NICU), imperative if your twins are born prematurely. However, some obstetricians also have advanced training in high-risk pregnancies so be sure to ask when you meet with one. Ultimately, who you decide to deliver your babies is a purely personal choice—like falling in love, you will just know it when you meet her. Your first step is making appointments and interviewing several possible candidates.

Questions to ask yourself:

- *How accessible is this obstetrician or perinatologist? Is his or her office close to home? Does he or she take my insurance?*

- *At which hospital does he or she have privileges? Does the hospital have a Level III NICU in case my babies are born prematurely?*

- *What kind of patient am I? Do I want to be a partner with my health-care provider or am I looking for someone who will guide me with lots of handing holding? And do my wishes mesh well with this doctor's personality?*

Questions to ask your obstetrician:

- *What is your philosophy on delivering twins? How many have you delivered vaginally in the past few years? How many by C-section? Which situation would warrant a C-section?*

- *Which tests and procedures do you routinely prescribe for moms carrying twins?*

- *What is your philosophy on the routine use of IVs, continuous fetal monitoring, or confinement to bed during labor?*

- *Do you use email to receive and answer questions?*

- *Who will deliver my babies if you are unavailable when I go into labor?*

Week 7

Pregnancy Tip

Early weight gain is key to a healthy twin pregnancy as it reduces the risk for preterm labor. Your goal? 24 pounds by Week 24. If you are of normal weight, you can reach that goal by consuming 3,000 to 3,500 calories with a minimum of 130 grams of protein each and every day.

30 WEEKS TO GO

Today's date: _____

My weight: _____

Pounds gained this week: _____

Pounds to go to reach my goal: _____

My growing waistline in inches: _____

My growing bust size in inches: _____

Questions to ask my doctor:

_____

_____

_____

_____

_____

My pregnancy symptoms:

_____

_____

_____

_____

_____

My Energy Level (circle one):   1   2   3   4   5

Moms Expecting Twins

A healthy diet is important for all moms expecting but for the mom pregnant with twins, it is doubly important as adequate weight gain helps to limit the possibility of preterm labor and premature delivery. Research shows a direct correlation between early maternal weight gain and strong fetal growth as it aids in the development and function of the placenta. Below is a sample menu that incorporates a healthy dose of both calories and protein. But consult your doctor first for his or her recommendations.

TOTAL CALORIES: 3,121   TOTAL GRAMS OF PROTEIN: 194

BREAKFAST

2 poached eggs *(140 calories/12 grams protein)*

2 slices of bacon *(160 calories/8 grams protein)*

2 slices whole-wheat toast with 2 tablespoons butter *(204 calories/7 grams protein)*

8 oz. glass of 2-percent milk *(130 calories/10 grams protein)*

MID-MORNING SNACK

¼ cup of almonds *(170 calories/7 grams protein)*

4 oz. whole-milk mozzarella *(340 calories/25 grams protein)*

1 tangerine/mandarin orange *(37 calories/0.6 grams protein)*

LUNCH

½ cup of tuna salad on whole-wheat toast *(332 calories/23.5 grams protein)*

½ cup red grapes *(52 calories/0.5 grams protein)*

8 oz. glass of 2-percent milk *(130 calories/10 grams protein)*

1 fun-size Almond Joy *(80 calories/1 gram protein)*

AFTERNOON SNACK

¼ cup hummus with 4-inch round, whole-wheat pita bread *(175 calories/7.5 grams protein)*

1 medium apple, sliced *(95 calories/0 protein)*

DINNER

Grilled chicken breast with skin *(280 calories/55 grams protein)*

½ cup brown rice with tablespoon of butter *(140 calories/2.5 grams protein)*

½ cup broccoli sautéed in 2 tablespoons olive oil *(127 calories/1.9 grams protein)*

8 oz. glass of 2-percent milk *(130 calories/10 grams protein)*

1 scoop (1/2 cup) vanilla ice cream *(145 calories/2.5 grams protein)*

BEDTIME SNACK

1 cup full-fat plain yogurt *(149 calories/9 grams protein)*

1 medium banana *(105 calories/1 gram protein)*

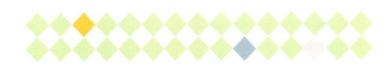

Week 8

My Baby Scan

Place Here

29 WEEKS TO GO

Today's date: _____

My weight: _____

Pounds gained this week: _____

Pounds to go to reach my goal: _____

My growing waistline in inches: _____

My growing bust size in inches: _____

Questions to ask my doctor:

_____
_____
_____
_____
_____

My pregnancy symptoms:

_____
_____
_____
_____
_____

My Energy Level (circle one):   1   2   3   4   5

Did You Know

that the incidence of spontaneous identical twinning (monozygotic) is about 1 in 250 pregnancies regardless of a mother's age, race or family history? However, women have a two to three times higher incidence of having identical twins following IVF (in-vitro fertilization). The reasons , however, are still not clear as to why it happens.

Twin Pregnancy
Food Diary

A healthy diet during a twin pregnancy is key but sometimes it can be difficult to know if you are getting enough calories and protein. That is why keeping a diary is a great idea. Just jot down your diet during the day and tally up your calories and grams of protein in the evening to see if you are on target to meeting your goal. On the following page is a sample diary. The template is also available at http://christinabaglivitinglof.com/free-download where you can download it for free. Print up a copy each day and tuck it in your handbag or briefcase to take it on the go. Below are a few tips to help make your food journal a success.

- *According to new guidelines, a woman pregnant with twins needs a minimum of 3,000 calories and 130 grams of protein each day. In addition, moms-to-be need extra folic acid (breads and cereal), calcium (dairy products like milk and cheese), and an abundance of iron (red meat, poultry, pork, and fish).*

- *To meet your daily caloric goal, shoot for three meals plus two to four snacks every day.*

- *Do not wait until you are famished before you eat. Instead "graze" throughout the day (keep snacks in your handbag or office desk) supplying your babies with a constant flow of nutrition. Added bonus? A full stomach curbs morning sickness.*

- *And do not forget to drink plenty of fluids! (Yes, women carrying twins require more fluids than women carrying singletons.) Water, juice, and milk are all good bets but coffee and tea, not so much. Shoot for at least ten, eight-ounce servings every day.*

MY FOOD DIARY NOTES

MY DAILY FOOD DIARY

Today's Date: _____

	WHAT DID I EAT TODAY?	CALORIE COUNT	GRAMS OF PROTEIN
BREAKFAST			
MID-MORNING SNACK			
LUNCH			
AFTERNOON SNACK			
DINNER			
BEDTIME SNACK			
MIDNIGHT			
	Daily Totals: (Try for 3,000 calories & 130 grams of protein each day.)		

Week 9

Place
My Baby-Bump
Photo here

Pregnancy Tip

Vegetarians expecting twins need to be extra vigilant about getting enough protein in their diets. Yet with careful meal planning, they can get an adequate amount. Legumes (beans, lentils, peanuts), tofu, nuts, dairy products (milk, yogurt, cheese), eggs, whole grains (quinoa, wheat germ, oat bran, wild rice) are all high in protein.

28 WEEKS TO GO

Today's date: _____

My weight: _____

Pounds gained this week: _____

Pounds to go to reach my goal: _____

My growing waistline in inches: _____

My growing bust size in inches: _____

Questions to ask my doctor:

_____
_____
_____
_____
_____

My pregnancy symptoms:

_____
_____
_____
_____
_____

My Energy Level (circle one):   1   2   3   4   5

Week: _____

Place
Baby "A's"
Ultrasound Photo
Here

Place
Baby "B's"
Ultrasound Photo
Here

Week 10

Place
My Baby-Bump
Photo Here

27 WEEKS TO GO

Today's date: _____

My weight: _____

Pounds gained this week: _____

Pounds to go to reach my goal: _____

My growing waistline in inches: _____

My growing bust size in inches: _____

Questions to ask my doctor:

_____
_____
_____
_____
_____

My pregnancy symptoms:

_____
_____
_____
_____
_____

My Energy Level (circle one):   1   2   3   4   5

Baby Budget Checklist

Surprises are fun but not if they are the financial kind! Take some of the sting out of the double ding to your family budget by making a plan before your twins arrive. To get started, use the checklist below as well as some great online tools by searching "baby cost calculators."

First Trimester: Weeks 6 to 12

☐ Set up a budget. Disposable diapers can run about $1,700 a year for two babies! (Cloth may be cheaper.) Formula will add another $2,500 a year (but breastfeeding is free).

☐ Pay off high-interest debt and sock away cash for a rainy day. Make a big effort to pay off those credit card bills before the babies arrive, and set aside money in an emergency fund. (Shoot for three months of living expenses, more if one parent plans to stay home full time.)

☐ Look into your childcare options. Depending on where you live, daycare or a private nanny can really take a bite out of your budget. Weigh the benefits of staying home against the cost of daycare.

☐ Call your insurance carrier to check on prenatal coverage. Budget for out-of-pocket medical costs such as co-pays and deductibles.

Second Trimester: Weeks 13 to 27

☐ Check on maternity leave policy with your employer. Does your company offer paid maternity leave? (Few companies do.) If not, see if you can use your accumulated sick days or vacation time to offset lost wages.

☐ Shop around for life insurance. Term life insurance offers the best bang for the buck. Search "term life insurance" online to compare rates.

☐ Set up a will or trust. If your estate is less than $2 million, your best option is the do-it-yourself route. At legalzoom.com, you can create a will online for about $100. The downloadable Quicken WillMaker Plus is even cheaper at $49.99.

☐ Designate a guardian for your twins. Choose someone who will love them fully and give them the attention they deserve. Here is a hint: A family member is not always the best choice.

Third Trimester: Weeks 28 to 37

☐ Scrutinize your baby register. To cut down on expenses, focus on your "needs" (double stroller, two car seats) and eliminate the "wants" (diaper genie, baby wipes warmer). Investigate borrowing big-ticket items such as cribs and accept all hand-me-down clothing.

☐ Open up individual 529 college savings plans for each twin. 529 plans offer tax-free growth and withdrawals for college. Many plans offer automatic monthly deductions of as little as $25 and some states allow tax breaks for contributions. Learn more at 529.com.

☐ Add twins to your health insurance. You have 30 days from the time of your twins' birth to add them to your policy otherwise you may have to wait until your next open enrollment.

☐ Think about upcoming tax season. Speak to your employer about adjusting your federal withholding to reflect your new family. For the 2015 tax year, the personal exemption is $4,000. Woo-hoo! That is $8,000 for twins! Furthermore, you can claim up to $1,000 per child under the Child Tax Credit (part of the American Taxpayer Relief Act of 2012).

Notes:

_____

_____

_____

_____

_____

_____

_____

_____

_____

Week 11

Did You Know

that if your twin pregnancy is complication free, you will visit your doctor once a month until Week 27, twice a month until week 34, then weekly until you deliver? You will have more ultrasounds, too—monthly beginning around Week 18 for moms expecting fraternal twins; more often for moms carrying identical twins.

26 WEEKS TO GO

Today's date: _____

My weight: _____

Pounds gained this week: _____

Pounds to go to reach my goal: _____

My growing waistline in inches: _____

My growing bust size in inches: _____

Questions to ask my doctor:

_____
_____
_____
_____
_____

My pregnancy symptoms:

_____
_____
_____
_____
_____

My Energy Level (circle one):   1   2   3   4   5

Today's Date: Sept 28, 2016

This is how we learned that we were expecting twins.

After 3 rounds of failed IUI's last years we decided to try IVF. On July 20, 2016 my eggs were retrieved and then fertilized for 5 days. On July 25, 2016 we placed the 2 strongest embryos back in my uterus. We were to wait 12 days for our first Beta test at Emory we couldn't wait that long. On Sunday, July 31, 2016 we took an at home pregnancy test. I was too scared to look so adam did. All I heard was "Why is the first line lighter then the second?" I of course lost it. I'd never seen a positive for us. we didn't get our hopes up since we were testing early but I was elated to say the least. No matter what happened from that moment I was a mom. we went for our Beta test as schedule on my 38th birthday, Aug 6, 2016. We were at adam's parents house. Hoping to get the official call before telling them. They were the only ones who didn't know we did IVF. The phone rings and we stepped into the spare room. My nurse Michelle says "Your numbers are 635!! How many embryos did we put back??" I said "2" She said "well I'm just going to let that sink in!" Every appt from their on out became more and more clear that you both decided to stick around and let us be your mommy + daddy and we couldn't be more excited! ♡♡

Week 12

Place
My Baby-Bump
Photo Here

Pregnancy Tip

If you are expecting identical twins, ask your obstetrician or perinatologist for a chorionicity scan. This ultrasound scan is important in determining if your twins share a placenta, a risk factor for twin-to-twin transfusion syndrome (TTTS). If they do share one placenta, you will be monitored more closely to help avoid future complications.

25 WEEKS TO GO

Today's date: _Sept 28, 2016_

My weight: _175_

Pounds gained this week: _____

Pounds to go to reach my goal: _____

My growing waistline in inches: _____

My growing bust size in inches: _____

Questions to ask my doctor:

Dry Skin
Migraines
Harmony test

My pregnancy symptoms:

Dry Skin, Migraines
Nausea, Shortness of
breath, back + neck
pain

My Energy Level (circle one):   1   2   ③   4   5

My Blood Pressure: _____

My Urine Screening Results: *Clear* _____

My Cervical Length: _____

Test Date: _____

Week Performed: _____

Name of Test: _____

Results: _____

Follow up needed? If so, where and when?

_____

Test Date: _____

Week Performed: _____

Name of Test: _____

Results: _____

Follow up needed? If so, where and when?

_____

Test Date: _____

Week Performed: _____

Name of Test: _____

Results: _____

Follow up needed? If so, where and when?

_____

Notes:

_____

_____

My Second Trimester

Week 13

Place My Baby-Bump Photo Here

24 WEEKS TO GO

Today's date: Oct 5, 2016

My weight: 178

Pounds gained this week: _____

Pounds to go to reach my goal: _____

My growing waistline in inches: _____

My growing bust size in inches: _____

Questions to ask my doctor:

_____
_____
_____
_____
_____

My pregnancy symptoms:

Nauseated, Migraines, Shortness of breath, mood swings, crying spells, dry skin, back pain

My Energy Level (circle one):   1   **2**   3   4   5

Maternity Clothes Shopping Tips

You'll need to start shopping for maternity clothes early in your second trimester. But before you drop some serious bucks on a new wardrobe, follow these tips to get the most out of your maternity clothes' budget.

- *First, see if you can borrow a few pieces from a former mom-to-be. If you score, jot down what you borrowed from whom so that you can return each item after your babies are born.*

- *To help keep costs down when you hit the mall, stick with basic separates that you can mix and match. Keep the color palate neutral concentrating on grey, black, and brown. If bold is your thing, accessorize your wardrobe with brightly colored or patterned scarves and belts.*

- *A-line and empire-waist dresses and shirts work well as they are not only flattering flowing away from your bust line but will fit you for most of your pregnancy.*

- *If you are on a budget, avoid maternity boutiques. There are plenty of inexpensive but trendy maternity designs available at Target and JCPenney.*

- *Think about the seasons. Will you be your biggest in summer or winter? Then plan your wardrobe accordingly as there is no use in buying a maternity swimsuit if you are due in spring.*

- *Avoid buying clothes that are merely a few sizes too large. They will hang oddly and not fit properly. To look your best, you need properly tailored maternity clothes.*

- *To make it easier for you, most designers size maternity clothing the same as regular clothing. So if you were a size 10 before pregnancy, look for size 10 in maternity clothing.*

- *Try everything on! It may take you twice as long but it is important nonetheless as no one wants to wear maternity clothes that don't fit properly.*

- *Most pregnant women's feet grow at least a half size. Do not forget to put shoes on the list!*

Maternity Clothes Wish List

TOPS

- ☐ T-Shirts
- ☐ Empire Blouses
- ☐ Tunics
- ☐ Cardigan

PANTS

- ☐ Leggings/Stretch Pants
- ☐ Dress Pants
- ☐ Jeans

SKIRTS/DRESSES

- ☐ Long Skirt with Elastic Waist
- ☐ Wrap Dress
- ☐ Empire Waist Dress

SLEEPWEAR

- ☐ Pajamas
- ☐ Robe

SEASONAL

- ☐ Swimsuit
- ☐ Holiday Dress
- ☐ Belted Coat

ACCESSORIES

- ☐ Belly Band
- ☐ Panties
- ☐ Support Hose
- ☐ Compression Socks
- ☐ Nursing Bra
- ☐ Flat Shoes

Shopping Tip:
Choose slip-on shoes (no bending over) a half size larger as your feet will grow.

Don't forget to dress in layers as moms-to-be go from hot to cold several times a day!

MY MATERNITY CLOTHES SHOPPING NOTES

Week 14

Place
My Baby-Bump
Photo Here

Did You Know

that it is OK to have sex during your twin pregnancy? Research has shown that as long as your pregnancy is progressing normally, lovemaking will not increase your chances of preterm labor. But err on the side of caution and speak with your doctor if you have concerns.

23 WEEKS TO GO

Today's date: 10-14-2016

My weight: 178.2

Pounds gained this week: _____

Pounds to go to reach my goal: _____

My growing waistline in inches: _____

My growing bust size in inches: _____

Questions to ask my doctor:

_____
_____
_____
_____
_____

My pregnancy symptoms:

_____
_____
_____
_____
_____

My Energy Level (circle one):   1   2   3   4   5

MY TWIN NURSERY PLANNING GRAPH

Use the graph below to sketch out your twins' nursery, playing around with furniture placement. Sketch with a pencil so that you can edit and refine your design as inspiration hits you.

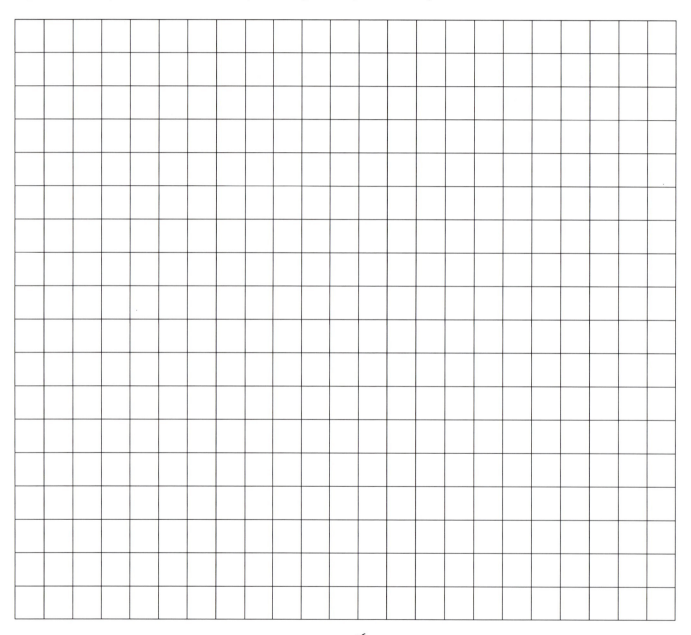

Place

Paint or

Fabric

Swatch Here

Place

Paint or

Fabric

Swatch Here

Place

Paint or

Fabric

Swatch Here

Place

Paint or

Fabric

Swatch Here

Place

Paint or

Fabric

Swatch Here

Place

Paint or

Fabric

Swatch Here

Place

Nursery Theme Idea

Photo Here

Place

Nursery Theme Idea

Photo Here

Place

Nursery Theme Idea

Photo Here

Place

Nursery Theme Idea

Photo Here

Twin Nursery
Furniture Checklist

It's time to start furnishing your twins' nursery. Below is a handy checklist to make sure they have everything that they need.

☐ Twin Bassinet: These days, you have several options when it comes to finding a bassinet specifically for twins (just Google it!). Try to find one that is portable.

☐ Crib: Yes, twins can share one for the first few months but you will need two by the time your twins hit month four to six. Furthermore, if you borrow that extra crib, make sure it meets current federal safety standards—the distance between slants should not be wider than 2 ⅜ inches. The mattress should be firm and at least six inches high (to help prevent SIDS, Sudden Infant Death Syndrome).

☐ Dresser: Opt for one that is 37 inches tall (counter height) so that you can easily add a changing pad on top.

☐ Changing Table/Table Top Pad: It is easy to forgo a changing table by simply buying a contoured changing pad and placing it on top of babies' dresser.

☐ Hamper: Convenient for dirty clothes; wicker baskets are a must for corralling baby stuff.

☐ Rocker/Glider/Armchair: It is a personal choice but a rocking chair can be an important accoutrement for late-night feedings and cuddling.

☐ Bookshelf/Storage: The toys and books will begin to flow into your nursery before you know it—be prepared with a spot to store them all neatly.

Week 15

Pregnancy Tip

Time to slow down! Getting off your feet reduces the pressure on your cervix and may help prevent preterm labor. Elevate your feet for 15 minutes several times a day, or better yet, lie down. If you can, try to lie on your left side as it takes the stress off your organs increasing blood flow (and nutrients) to your babies.

22 WEEKS TO GO

Today's date: _____

My weight: _____

Pounds gained this week: _____

Pounds to go to reach my goal: _____

My growing waistline in inches: _____

My growing bust size in inches: _____

Questions to ask my doctor:

_____

_____

_____

_____

_____

My pregnancy symptoms:

_____

_____

_____

_____

_____

My Energy Level (circle one): 1 2 3 4 5

Today's Date: _____

This is how we shared the news with family and friends.

_____

_____

_____

_____

_____

_____

_____

_____

_____

_____

_____

_____

_____

_____

_____

_____

_____

_____

_____

_____

_____

Week 16

Place
My Baby Bump
Photo Here

Pregnancy Tip

Resting fully reclined during the day is great for your babies but avoid sleeping on your back at night as it puts pressure on a major blood vessel, decreasing blood flow to your babies. Instead try sleeping on your side (preferably your left side), using a body pillow for support.

21 WEEKS TO GO

Today's date: _____

My weight: _____

Pounds gained this week: _____

Pounds to go to reach my goal: _____

My growing waistline in inches: _____

My growing bust size in inches: _____

Questions to ask my doctor:

_____
_____
_____
_____
_____

My pregnancy symptoms:

_____
_____
_____
_____
_____

My Energy Level (circle one):   1   2   3   4   5

Week: _____

Place

Baby "A's"

Ultrasound Photo

Here

Place

Baby "B's"

Ultrasound Photo

Here

Week: _____

Place
Baby "A's"
Ultrasound Photo
Here

Place
Baby "B's"
Ultrasound Photo
Here

MY TWIN PREGNANCY

Week 17

Did You Know

that even if you are confined to bed rest during your pregnancy that you can still have a baby shower? You actually have several options: You can wait until after the babies are born (your guests would love to see your babies) or let your guests come to your bedside! If you are in the hospital, you can even hold your shower remotely via Skype, FaceTime or webcam. (So be sure to create your baby registry early, just in case!)

20 WEEKS TO GO

Today's date: _____

My weight: _____

Pounds gained this week: _____

Pounds to go to reach my goal: _____

My growing waistline in inches: _____

My growing bust size in inches: _____

Questions to ask my doctor:

_____

_____

_____

_____

_____

My pregnancy symptoms:

_____

_____

_____

_____

_____

My Energy Level (circle one):   1   2   3   4   5

MY TWIN BABY SHOWER

So when is the party? A twin baby shower is double the fun! Ask your hostess to schedule the big day no later than Week 28 just in case your babies decide to make an early entrance.

GUEST LIST

_____	_____	_____
_____	_____	_____
_____	_____	_____
_____	_____	_____
_____	_____	_____
_____	_____	_____
_____	_____	_____
_____	_____	_____

Twin Registry "Must Haves"

Week 18

Place
My Baby-Bump
Photo Here

19 WEEKS TO GO

Today's date: _____

My weight: _____

Pounds gained this week: _____

Pounds to go to reach my goal: _____

My growing waistline in inches: _____

My growing bust size in inches: _____

Questions to ask my doctor:

_____

_____

_____

_____

_____

My pregnancy symptoms:

_____

_____

_____

_____

_____

My Energy Level (circle one):   1   2   3   4   5

MY LATEST TEST RESULTS

My Blood Pressure: _____

My Urine Screening Results: _____

My Cervical Length: _____

Test Date: _____   Results: _____

Week Performed: _____   Follow up needed? If so, where and when?

Name of Test: _____   _____

Test Date: _____   Results: _____

Week Performed: _____   Follow up needed? If so, where and when?

Name of Test: _____   _____

Test Date: _____   Results: _____

Week Performed: _____   Follow up needed? If so, where and when?

Name of Test: _____   _____

Notes:

_____

_____

Week 19

Place
My Baby-Bump
Photo Here

18 WEEKS TO GO

Today's date: _____

My weight: _____

Pounds gained this week: _____

Pounds to go to reach my goal: _____

My growing waistline in inches: _____

My growing bust size in inches: _____

Questions to ask my doctor:

_____

_____

_____

_____

_____

My pregnancy symptoms:

_____

_____

_____

_____

_____

My Energy Level (circle one):   1   2   3   4   5

Tips to Choosing a
Childbirth Class

Some moms expecting twins skip taking a childbirth class believing that since they will end up having a C-section, why bother. Should you skip it, too? Absolutely not. While it is true that nearly 50 percent of moms carrying twins have a cesarean, you may not be one of them. Furthermore, a good childbirth class offers much more than just teaching you how to pant and breathe! A good class takes the mystery out of the birthing process, and helps you build confidence in your body, lessening your anxiety as delivery approaches. Finally, childbirth class discusses a whole host of pregnancy as well as post-partum topics including baby care. But to have a positive experience, you will need to choose the right class. Here are a few guidelines to get you started.

- *Sign up early. Not only could your babies show up before Week 37, you could be put on bed rest. Plus, attending class earlier rather than later allows you to practice and implement all that you have learned. Begin your classes around Week 20 but no later than Week 24.*

- *Choose a class where the instructor is a licensed medical professional or has completed a recognized course in childbirth education. In addition, find out how much experience the instructor has with multiple births—twins, triplets, and well as quads.*

- *Ask if topics covered include information specific to multiples, such as cesarean delivery.*

- *Make sure the class philosophy matches your personal beliefs. There are many different types of childbirth classes out there: Lamaze, Bradley, and Hypnobirthing, to name a few. Each has its own point of view when it comes to such topics as the use of pain medication during labor.*

- *Class size does matter. A smaller class allows for plenty of group discussion and a chance to get to know the other parents in your group.*

- *Look for a birthing class specifically for moms expecting multiples. Yes, they do exist, although most are one-day seminars to be taken along with a regular childbirth class. Call around to local hospitals to see if they have classes specifically geared towards couples expecting multiples.*

Week 20

Pregnancy Tip

Ask your obstetrician or perinatologist for a vaginal ultrasound around Week 20 to check the length of your cervix. Then ask for a follow-up ultrasound four weeks later. Studies have shown that if your cervical length (CL) shortens by 13 percent or more by the second scan, you are at risk for preterm labor and should be monitored more closely.

17 WEEKS TO GO

Today's date: _____

My weight: _____

Pounds gained this week: _____

Pounds to go to reach my goal: _____

My growing waistline in inches: _____

My growing bust size in inches: _____

Questions to ask my doctor:

_____

_____

_____

_____

_____

My pregnancy symptoms:

_____

_____

_____

_____

_____

My Energy Level (circle one):   1   2   3   4   5

Tips to Naming Twins

Choosing names for your twins is a challenge. A fun challenge but a challenge nonetheless. For some couples, agreeing on one name is difficult enough, but two? Yikes! Have fun with the process but remember that the names you choose will be with your children their entire lives (but, hey, no pressure). Here is what to consider before you name your future presidents.

- *Twins go through their childhood as a pair so you may want to choose two completely different names to help stress their individuality.*

- *Some twins look so alike that similar sounding, alliterated names such as David and Daniel or Mason and Marshall might further confuse family and friends. Furthermore, they already have the same last name and the same birthday—having the same first initial could cause a mix up with public records during the school years and beyond.*

- *If you want their names to complement each other, however, consider matching syllable count (such as the two-syllable names, Gavin and Emma) or names that have similar endings (such as the "ia" in Mia and Sophia). Or, if you are really clever with words, try using anagrams of each other as in Anise and Siena, or Isabel and Blaise.*

- *Choose names that will withstand the test of time. And before you commit, try to visualize your twins as adults. Will they thank you for naming them Chance and Chase, or will they be heading to court to have them changed?*

GIRL-GIRL NAMES

_____   _____

_____   _____

_____   _____

_____   _____

_____   _____

_____   _____

BOY-BOY NAMES

_____   _____

_____   _____

_____   _____

_____   _____

_____   _____

_____   _____

_____   _____

_____   _____

_____   _____

_____   _____

_____   _____

_____   _____

_____   _____

OUR TOP THREE COMBINATIONS

_____   _____

_____

Week 21

Place
My Baby Bump
Photo Here

16 WEEKS TO GO

Today's date: _____

My weight: _____

Pounds gained this week: _____

Pounds to go to reach my goal: _____

My growing waistline in inches: _____

My growing bust size in inches: _____

Questions to ask my doctor:

_____
_____
_____
_____
_____

My pregnancy symptoms:

_____
_____
_____
_____
_____

My Energy Level (circle one):   1   2   3   4   5

Know the
Signs of Preeclampsia

Did you know that women expecting twins are at a much higher risk for developing preeclampsia, a serious pregnancy condition marked by a rapid rise in blood pressure combined with excessive protein in the urine? (Moms expecting singletons run a five to eight percent risk of developing the condition while mothers pregnant with twins have a 25 to 30 percent chance.) Preeclampsia usually occurs sometime after Week 20 and if left untreated it could lead to potentially fatal eclampsia. No one wants to hear that (especially moms pregnant with twins) but knowledge is power! The good news is if caught early, moms can go on to deliver healthy babies and recover fully. But much like preterm labor, the signs of preeclampsia are often subtle. Many moms dismiss symptoms, thinking it is all part of general pregnancy discomfort. But not you! You listen to your body, and you will call your doctor immediately if you have any of these symptoms, right?

- *Hands, feet, and especially face and ankles become excessively puffy.*

- *A headache that just will not go away.*

- *A change in eyesight: blurry vision including seeing "spots," and sensitivity to light.*

- *Nausea or vomiting.*

- *Abdominal pain in the upper right corner of chest, similar to heartburn. Or, shoulder pain.*

- *Shortness of breath, rapid heartbeat, or general feeling of confusion.*

- *Rapid weight gain of nearly a pound or more per day.*

Week 22

Place
My Baby Bump
Photo Here

Pregnancy Tip

You can limit your risk of preeclampsia by keeping all prenatal appointments where your blood pressure will be closely monitored. Furthermore, concentrate on high-fiber foods and calcium as studies suggest that both may help reduce your risk. And finally, stay away from processed food as they are often high in sodium, a contributing factor to hypertension.

15 WEEKS TO GO

Today's date: _____

My weight: _____

Pounds gained this week: _____

Pounds to go to reach my goal: _____

My growing waistline in inches: _____

My growing bust size in inches: _____

Questions to ask my doctor:

_____
_____
_____
_____
_____

My pregnancy symptoms:

_____
_____
_____
_____
_____

My Energy Level (circle one):　　1　　2　　3　　4　　5

CAR SEAT COMPARISON CHART

	CAR SEAT #1	CAR SEAT #2	CAR SEAT #3	CAR SEAT #4
BRAND & MODEL #				
SEAT TYPE: INFANT, CONVERTIBLE, BOOSTER				
WEIGHT/WIDTH				
COST				
STORE WITH BEST PRICE				
Rate Qualities Below: 1 to 5	Rate Qualities Below: 1 to 5	Rate Qualities Below: 1 to 5	Rate Qualities Below: 1 to 5	Rate Qualities Below: 1 to 5
EASE OF USE				
EASE OF CLEANING				
PADDING & HEAD SUPPORT				
CRASH PROTECTION RATING				

Download a free Car Seat Comparison Chart: http:// christinabaglivitinglof.com/free-download

Week 23

Place
My Baby-Bump
Photo Here

Pregnant Tip

If you find yourself waking in the middle of the night ravenous, it is a good sign as it means your babies are growing rapidly. To combat your midnight hunger pains, try a calcium-rich snack before bed as the fat breaks down more slowly, or keep a little snack tray of cheese and crackers by your bedside and take a few bites when heading to the bathroom to pee.

14 WEEKS TO GO

Today's date: _____

My weight: _____

Pounds gained this week: _____

Pounds to go to reach my goal: _____

My growing waistline in inches: _____

My growing bust size in inches: _____

Questions to ask my doctor:

_____
_____
_____
_____
_____

My pregnancy symptoms:

_____
_____
_____
_____
_____

My Energy Level (circle one):   1   2   3   4   5

Know the
Signs of Preterm Labor

The biggest worry for moms expecting twins—by far—is the fear of going into labor before their due date. (By definition, preterm labor occurs prior to Week 37.) And with due cause as approximately only 40 percent of women carrying twins make it to Week 37. Yet did you know that if labor is caught in time (the cervix has not dilated past two centimeters and the amniotic sacs have not ruptured) labor can be stopped with medication? The key is to know the signs of preterm labor and alert your doctor immediately. Yet the beginning signs of labor are often subtle, leaving many moms-to-be wondering and confused. Your best defense? Educate yourself on the signs of preterm labor and do not hesitate to call your doctor if you think you may be in labor. If you experience any of the symptoms below, call your doctor. You will not be bothering her; she will not think that you are overreacting. Just call her.

- *Menstrual-like cramps with or without diarrhea.*

- *Upset stomach or vomiting.*

- *Six or more contractions per hour.* **Or,** *contractions that increase in frequency.*

- *Strong pelvic pressure.*

- *A dull, low backache.*

- *Or, pain radiating from your upper thighs.*

- *Change in vaginal discharge, especially if it is bloody or watery.*

- *Just an innate sense that "something isn't right."*

Week 24

13 WEEKS TO GO

Did You Know

that women expecting twins are more likely to develop gestational diabetes than women carrying singletons? Your risk increases if you are over 30, were overweight at the start of your pregnancy, or have a family history. Your doctor will screen for glucose in your urine at every visit, and order a glucose tolerance test around Week 24 to determine if you have the condition. (Good news: It can be treated through diet.)

Today's date: _____

My weight: _____

Pounds gained this week: _____

Pounds to go to reach my goal: _____

My growing waistline in inches: _____

My growing bust size in inches: _____

Questions to ask my doctor:

_____

_____

_____

_____

_____

My pregnancy symptoms:

_____

_____

_____

_____

_____

My Energy Level (circle one):   1   2   3   4   5

My Blood Pressure: _____

My Urine Screening Results: _____

My Cervical Length: _____

Test Date: _____

Week Performed: _____

Name of Test: _____

Results: _____

Follow up needed? If so, where and when?

_____

Test Date: _____

Week Performed: _____

Name of Test: _____

Results: _____

Follow up needed? If so, where and when?

_____

Test Date: _____

Week Performed: _____

Name of Test: _____

Results: _____

Follow up needed? If so, where and when?

_____

Notes:

_____

_____

Week 25

Place
My Baby-Bump
Photo Here

Did You Know

that you reached an important milestone? It is "viability." If your twins are born this week, they have a good chance of survival. They will still spend several months in the NICU, of course, but their long-term prognosis is good. So try to relax and enjoy the remaining weeks of your twin pregnancy (but continue to concentrate on protein in your diet).

12 WEEKS TO GO

Today's date: _____

My weight: _____

Pounds gained this week: _____

Pounds to go to reach my goal: _____

My growing waistline in inches: _____

My growing bust size in inches: _____

Questions to ask my doctor:

_____
_____
_____
_____
_____

My pregnancy symptoms:

_____
_____
_____
_____
_____

My Energy Level (circle one):   1   2   3   4   5

DOUBLE STROLLER COMPARISON CHART

	STROLLER #1	STROLLER #2	STROLLER #3	STROLLER #4
BRAND & MODEL #				
STROLLER TYPE				
WEIGHT & WIDTH				
COST				
Rate Qualities Below, 1 - 5	Rate Qualities Below, 1 - 5	Rate Qualities Below, 1 - 5	Rate Qualities Below, 1 - 5	Rate Qualities Below, 1 - 5
EASE OF OPENING/CLOSING				
SEAT ADJUSTMENT & DEGREE OF RECLINE				
HANDLING: MANEUVERING & CORNERING				
EXTRAS: CUP HOLDERS, BASKETS, ETC.				

Download a free Double Stroller Comparison Chart: http://christinabaglivitinglof.com/free-download

Week 26

My Baby-Bump Photo Here

Pregnancy Tip

When writing up your birth plan, be sure to include these different scenarios: vaginal birth, cesarean birth, and vaginal followed by cesarean. All three are possible outcomes for the mom about to give birth to twins. If you have your preferences in writing, however, there's less of a chance for surprises. (Although you should review your plan with your health-care provider just in case.)

11 WEEKS TO GO

Today's Date: _____

My weight: _____

Pounds gained this week: _____

Pounds to go to reach my goal: _____

My growing waistline in inches: _____

My growing bust size in inches: _____

Questions to ask my doctor:

_____
_____
_____
_____
_____

My pregnancy symptoms:

_____
_____
_____
_____
_____

My Energy Level (circle one):   1   2   3   4   5

Week: _____

Place
Baby "A's"
Ultrasound Photo
Here

Place
Baby "B's"
Ultrasound Photo
Here

Week 27

Did You Know

that nearly 15 percent of fraternal twins are in fact identical? Researchers speculate that there is a lack of knowledge among the medical community in understanding that nearly 25 percent of identical twins have separate placentas! There are a few ways to tell if your twins are identical such as prenatal amniocentesis or a DNA blood test after the twins are born.

10 WEEKS TO GO

Today's date: _____

My weight: _____

Pounds gained this week: _____

Pounds to go to reach my goal: _____

My growing waistline in inches: _____

My growing bust size in inches: _____

Questions to ask my doctor:

_____
_____
_____
_____
_____

My pregnancy symptoms:

_____
_____
_____
_____
_____

My Energy Level (circle one):   1   2   3   4   5

Today's Date: _____

Let me tell you about my wildly changing body.

_____
_____
_____
_____
_____
_____
_____
_____
_____
_____
_____
_____
_____
_____
_____
_____
_____
_____
_____
_____

My Third Trimester

MY TWIN PREGNANCY

Week 28

Did You Know

that Multiples of America (formerly known as The National Organization of Mothers of Twins Clubs) boasts the largest network of parents of multiples clubs in the world? Joining your local club is a wonderful way to connect with other moms with twins. Find a club in your area at nomotc.org.

9 WEEKS TO GO

Today's date: _____

My weight: _____

Pounds gained this week: _____

Pounds to go to reach my goal: _____

My growing waistline in inches: _____

My growing bust size in inches: _____

Questions to ask my doctor:

_____

_____

_____

_____

_____

My pregnancy symptoms:

_____

_____

_____

_____

_____

My Energy Level (circle one):   1   2   3   4   5

My Blood Pressure: _____

My Urine Screening Results: _____

My Cervical Length: _____

Test Date: _____   Results: _____

Week Performed: _____   Follow up needed? If so, where and when?

Name of Test: _____   _____

Test Date: _____   Results: _____

Week Performed: _____   Follow up needed? If so, where and when?

Name of Test: _____   _____

Test Date: _____   Results: _____

Week Performed: _____   Follow up needed? If so, where and when?

Name of Test: _____   _____

Notes:

_____

_____

Week 29

Place
My Baby Bump
Photo Here

8 WEEKS TO GO

Today's date: _____

My weight: _____

Pounds gained this week: _____

Pounds to go to reach my goal: _____

My growing waistline in inches: _____

My growing bust size in inches: _____

Questions to ask my doctor:

_____

_____

_____

_____

_____

My pregnancy symptoms:

_____

_____

_____

_____

_____

My Energy Level (circle one):   1   2   3   4   5

MY POST TWINS HELP SCHEDULE

Week of _____

	Sunday	Monday	Tuesday	Wednesday	Thursday	Friday	Saturday
7 a.m.							
8 a.m.							
9 a.m.							
10 a.m.							
11 a.m.							
NOON							
1 p.m.							
2 p.m.							
3 p.m.							
4 p.m.							
5 p.m.							
6 p.m.							
7 p.m.							
8 p.m.							
9 p.m.							
10 p.m.							
11 p.m.							

Download a free Post Twins Help Schedule: http://christinabaglivitinglof.com/free-download

Week 30

Pregnancy Tip

Stretch marks are not inevitable even for moms expecting twins! Heredity plays a role, as does the use of certain medications such as corticosteroid. Postpartum laser therapy, microdermabrasion, and tretinoin cream have all proven somewhat successful in diminishing the appearance of stretch marks.

7 WEEKS TO GO

Today's date: _____

My weight: _____

Pounds gained this week: _____

Pounds to go to reach my goal: _____

My growing waistline in inches: _____

My growing bust size in inches: _____

Questions to ask my doctor:

_____
_____
_____
_____
_____

My pregnancy symptoms:

_____
_____
_____
_____
_____

My Energy Level (circle one):　　1　　2　　3　　4　　5

Dear Baby "A":

Today's Date: _____

_____

_____

_____

_____

_____

_____

_____

_____

_____

_____

_____

_____

_____

_____

_____

_____

_____

Love, Mom

Dear Baby "B":   Today's Date: _____

_____

_____

_____

_____

_____

_____

_____

_____

_____

_____

_____

_____

_____

_____

_____

_____

_____

_____

Love, Mom

Week 31

Place
My Baby Bump
Photo Here

Pregnancy Tip

Be sure to tour the NICU of the hospital where you will be delivering. If your babies are born prior to Week 37, they will most likely spend some time there (depending on when they arrive, it could be as short as just a few days to several months). Getting yourself acquainted with the procedures and sounds of the NICU will help alleviate your anxiety.

6 WEEKS TO GO

Today's date: _____

My weight: _____

Pounds gained this week: _____

Pounds to go to reach my goal: _____

My growing waistline in inches: _____

My growing bust size in inches: _____

Questions to ask my doctor:

_____

_____

_____

_____

_____

My pregnancy symptoms:

_____

_____

_____

_____

_____

My Energy Level (circle one):   1   2   3   4   5

Dear Babies:

Today's Date: _____

_____

_____

_____

_____

_____

_____

_____

_____

_____

_____

_____

_____

_____

_____

_____

_____

_____

_____

_____

Love, Dad

Week 32

Place
My Baby Bump
Photo Here

5 WEEKS TO GO

Today's date: _____

My weight: _____

Pounds gained this week: _____

Pounds to go to reach my goal: _____

My growing waistline in inches: _____

My growing bust size in inches: _____

Questions to ask my doctor:

_____
_____
_____
_____
_____

My pregnancy symptoms:

_____
_____
_____
_____
_____

My Energy Level (circle one):   1   2   3   4   5

MY LATEST TEST RESULTS

My Blood Pressure: _____

My Urine Screening Results: _____

My Cervical Length: _____

Test Date: _____

Week Performed: _____

Name of Test: _____

Results: _____

Follow up needed? If so, where and when?

_____

Test Date: _____

Week Performed: _____

Name of Test: _____

Results: _____

Follow up needed? If so, where and when?

_____

Test Date: _____

Week Performed: _____

Name of Test: _____

Results: _____

Follow up needed? If so, where and when?

_____

Notes:

_____

_____

Week 33

Place
My Baby-Bump
Photo Here

4 WEEKS TO GO

Today's date: _____

My weight: _____

Pounds gained this week: _____

Pounds to go to reach my goal: _____

My growing waistline in inches: _____

My growing bust size in inches: _____

Questions to ask my doctor:

_____

_____

_____

_____

_____

My pregnancy symptoms:

_____

_____

_____

_____

_____

My Energy Level (circle one):   1   2   3   4   5

Twin Layette Checklist

Your twins are almost here! Now is the time to make sure your nursery is in order so you will have everything you need once your babies are home. But don't bombard your home with lots of "baby paraphernalia." During the first six months, your twins don't require much more than you. With that said, here are the essentials.

Nursery Bedding

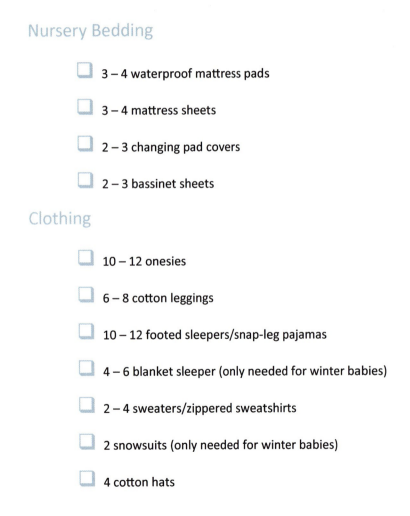

- ☐ 3 – 4 waterproof mattress pads
- ☐ 3 – 4 mattress sheets
- ☐ 2 – 3 changing pad covers
- ☐ 2 – 3 bassinet sheets

Clothing

- ☐ 10 – 12 onesies
- ☐ 6 – 8 cotton leggings
- ☐ 10 – 12 footed sleepers/snap-leg pajamas
- ☐ 4 – 6 blanket sleeper (only needed for winter babies)
- ☐ 2 – 4 sweaters/zippered sweatshirts
- ☐ 2 snowsuits (only needed for winter babies)
- ☐ 4 cotton hats

- ☐ 2 sets of booties or soft-bottom shoes
- ☐ 10 – 12 pairs of socks
- ☐ 24 burp cloths
- ☐ 10 – 12 bibs
- ☐ 8 – 10 cotton swaddling blankets
- ☐ 2 – 4 wool blankets (for stroller, not crib)
- ☐ 2 – 4 hooded bath towels
- ☐ 2 – 4 infant washcloths

Gear

- ☐ 2 rear-facing car seats
- ☐ double stroller
- ☐ port-a-crib
- ☐ 2 vibrating bouncy seats
- ☐ nursing pillow (if breastfeeding)
- ☐ 20 - 24, 8 oz. bottles (if bottle feeding)
- ☐ baby monitor
- ☐ plush changing pad
- ☐ changing station organizer (to stow baby wipes, diapers, cotton balls, etc.)

After Month Six

Now the real fun begins. Your twins are more active, more engaging as many twins are now on the go, crawling about discovering their surroundings. Now is the time to get that second crib (if you haven't already done so) plus some additional gear to help with getting you out of the house with your twins.

Nursery Bedding (for the second crib)

☐ 2 – 3 waterproof mattress pads

☐ 2 – 3 fitted mattress sheets

Gear

☐ 1 – 2 baby backpack

☐ 1 – 2 baby sling

☐ 2 umbrella strollers

☐ 2 high chairs or portable hook-on high chairs ("tot lock")

☐ activity gym

☐ superyard

Twin Layette Notes:

_____

_____

Week 34

Place
My Baby Bump
Photo Here

Did You Know

that the "presentation," or the position of your twins in your uterus, will determine your chances of having a cesarean or a vaginal delivery? If both babies are head down—in approximately 40% of twin pregnancies—chances for vaginal delivery are good. (But familiarize yourself with what goes on during a cesarean delivery just in case.)

3 WEEKS TO GO

Today's date: _____

My weight: _____

Pounds gained this week: _____

Pounds to go to reach my goal: _____

My growing waistline in inches: _____

My growing bust size in inches: _____

Questions to ask my doctor:

_____
_____
_____
_____
_____

My pregnancy symptoms:

_____
_____
_____
_____
_____

My Energy Level (circle one):   1   2   3   4   5

Place
Sample Announcement #1
Here

Place
Sample Announcement #2
Here

Birth Announcement Wording:

_____

_____

_____

_____

_____

Week 35

Place
My Baby-Bump
Photo Here

2 WEEKS TO GO

Did You Know

that even non-identical (or fraternal) twins can be difficult to tell apart in the first few weeks following birth? To avoid confusion, have a system in place to distinguish Twin "A" from Twin "B." For instance, paint one toenail on each baby a different color, or keep babies' hospital bracelets on until you are sure you can tell them apart.

Today's date: _____

My weight: _____

Pounds gained this week: _____

Pounds to go to reach my goal: _____

My growing waistline in inches: _____

My growing bust size in inches: _____

Questions to ask my doctor:

_____

_____

_____

_____

_____

My pregnancy symptoms:

_____

_____

_____

_____

_____

My Energy Level (circle one):   1   2   3   4   5

MY BABY SHOWER MEMORIES

The baby shower was held on _____

The shower was hosted by _____

The shower was held at

_____

The menu included

_____

_____

The party theme was

_____

_____

The decorations included

_____

_____

The cake was

_____

I was most surprised when

_____

_____

It was so funny when

_____

_____

My gifts included

_____

_____

Place

Baby Shower

Photo Here

Place

Baby Shower

Photo Here

Place

Baby Shower

Photo Here

Place

Baby Shower

Photo Here

Week 36

Place
My Baby-Bump
Photo Here

1 WEEK TO GO

Did You Know

that studies have shown that labor is slower for women carrying twins? Since the uterus is overly stretched, it doesn't contract as efficiently. (So don't let your doctor be so quick in calling "failure to progress.") Yet twins are usually born smaller than full-term singleton babies so delivery may be easier. (Now doesn't that sound nice?)

Today's date: _____

My weight: _____

Pounds gained this week: _____

Pounds to go to reach my goal: _____

My growing waistline in inches: _____

My growing bust size in inches: _____

Questions to ask my doctor:

_____
_____
_____
_____
_____

My pregnancy symptoms:

_____
_____
_____
_____
_____

My Energy Level (circle one):   1   2   3   4   5

DAILY FEEDING & DIAPERING CHART

Today's Date: _____

Twin "A" _____   Twin "B" _____

Time	Minutes Nursed or CC of Formula	L/R Side Nursed	Pee/ Poop	Nap	Bath	Meds and Notes

Time	Minutes Nursed or CC of Formula	L/R Side Nursed	Pee/ Poop	Nap	Bath	Meds and Notes

Week 37

Place
My Baby-Bump
Photo Here

IT'S TIME!

Today's date: _____

My weight: _____

Pounds gained this week: _____

Pounds to go to reach my goal: _____

My growing waistline in inches: _____

My growing bust size in inches: _____

Questions to ask my doctor:

_____

_____

_____

_____

_____

My pregnancy symptoms:

_____

_____

_____

_____

_____

My Excitement Level! (circle one):   1   2   3   4   5

Today's Date: _____

This is the story of the day you were born.

_____

_____

_____

_____

_____

_____

_____

_____

_____

_____

_____

_____

_____

_____

_____

_____

_____

_____

_____

_____

_____

_____

My Newborn Twins

Place
Baby "A"
Photo Here

Baby "A" was born on: _____

Baby "A" arrived at _____ am/pm

Baby "A" weighed: _____

Baby "A's" length: _____

Baby "A" looks like _____

And Baby "A's" name is

_____

Baby "B" was born on: _____

Baby "B" arrived at _____ am/pm

Baby "B" weighed: _____

Baby "B's" length: _____

Baby "B" looks like _____

And Baby "B's" name is

_____

Place
Baby "B"
Photo Here

Place

Twin A's Footprint

Here

Place

Twin B's Footprint

Here

55043976R00069

Made in the USA
Lexington, KY
07 September 2016